ISBN 978-0-331-06955-6
PIBN 11010287

ON

MILITARY HYGIENE

AND

THERAPEUTICS.

REPORT OF COMMITTEE ON MILITARY SURGERY TO THE SURGICAL SECTION OF THE NEW YORK ACADEMY OF MEDICINE.

FOURTH EDITION.

PRINTED FOR CIRCULATION BY
THE UNITED STATES SANITARY COMMISSION.
1865.

THE attention of The United States Sanitary Commission has been directed to the fact, that most of our Army Surgeons, now in the field, are unavoidably deprived of many facilities they have heretofore enjoyed for the consultation of standard medical authorities. It is obviously impossible to place within their reach any thing that can be termed a medical library. The only remedy seems to be the preparation and distribution among the medical staff, of a series of brief essays or hand-books, embodying, in a condensed form, the conclusions of the highest medical authorities in regard to those medical and surgical questions which are likely to present themselves to surgeons in the field, on the largest scale, and which are, therefore, of chief practical importance.

The Commission has assigned the duty of preparing papers on several subjects of this nature, to certain of its associate members, in our principal cities, belonging to the medical profession, whose names are the best evidence of their fitness for their duty.

The following paper on "Military Hygiene and Therapeutics" belongs to this series, and is respectfully recommended by the Commission to the medical officers of our army now in the field.

FRED. LAW OLMSTED,
Secretary.

WASHINGTON, June 21, 1861.

MILITARY HYGIENE

AND

THERAPEUTICS.

Your Committee begs leave respectfully to report that it has directed its attention chiefly to matters of practical interest which are not discussed in the ordinary books on surgery. The duties of a military surgeon involve a high degree of responsibility, and upon their skilful and faithful performance, the efficiency and success of armies is largely dependent. The ancient poet took a correct but altogether too limited view of the usefulness of military surgeons, when he uttered the sentiment—

> "A wise physician, skilled our wounds to heal,
> Is more than armies to the public weal."

The principal duties of the medical staff of the army are comprehended in the two classes of military hygiene and military therapeutics. The former of these two classes, although it attracts much less popular attention than the latter, is by no means inferior to it in practical importance. The statistics of armies clearly reveal the fact, that a much larger number of soldiers die from disease, resulting from unfavorable hygienic circumstances, than from wounds inflicted in battle. Even the dreadful slaughter of Waterloo and Solferino has been exceeded in its desolating power by the pestilential diseases by which large armies have sometimes been invaded. A few examples will suffice to show the extent to which armies have been scourged by disease. Sir David Stewart mentions "that the 92d regiment lost more officers and men in four months from the climate of Jamaica, than by the hand of the enemy in an active war of 22 years, in the progress of which it was 26 times in battle." Sir James McGrigor, in his account of the diseases of the Peninsular army in 1812, 1813, and a part of 1814, says "that there were 68,894 cases of fever, of which 6,703 died, equal to 9.7 per cent.; and 7,526 cases of dysentery, of which 4,717 died, equal to 62.5 per cent." Sir John Pringle says, "that of the troops stationed, during 1847, in South Beviland and the Island of Walcheren, some of the corps were so sickly as not to have more than one hundred men fit for duty, which was less than the seventh part of a complete battalion." In a paper by Mr. Edmonds, compiled from returns in the Adjutant-general's Office, it is stated that "in the Peninsular army, averaging a strength of 64,227, including officers and men, the annual ratio of mortality, from the 25th December, 1810, to 25th of May, 1813, was 10 per cent. of the officers, and 16 per cent. of the men, and that this army had during the above period 22½ per cent. constantly sick." In the report of the British Sanitary Commission dispatched to the seat of war in the East, in 1856, it is stated that "on the week ending April 7th, the sick and wounded amounted to 124 in every thousand, or nearly an eighth part of the army. The wounded were only five per cent. of this proportion. The force amounted to 31,610 men." After the attack on the Redan, the wounds amounted to 40 per cent. of the admissions, the remaining 60 per cent. being sick. During ten weeks, the admissions from wounds amounted to 3,858, or ten per cent. of the force; and the deaths from wounds to 334=0.37 per cent. of the force. During the same period, the admissions for disease amounted to 18,683=48.7 per cent. of the force, and deaths from disease to 1,309=3.04 per cent. of the force, or at the rate of 17.6 per cent. per annum. Only 17 per cent. of the total admissions, and 20 per cent. of the total deaths, were due to wounds exclusive of deaths on the field. Bazancourt, in his account of the Expedition to the Crimea, speaking of the operations in the Dobrudscha, says that "General Yusuf had resolved by a night march to fall suddenly upon the body of troops assembled around Babadagh, but at the moment when (at about 6 o'clock in the evening) the order for departure was given, 500 men lay stretched upon the earth unable to rise: the cholera had fallen like a thunder-bolt upon the expeditionary column. At 8 o'clock, there were already 150 dead, and 350 dying." The pestilence continued its ravages, and the expedition to the Dobrudscha was consequently given up.

The whole number of officers and men sent to the East by the French government, during the period of two years, was 309,268. Of this number 200,000 were under treatment at the ambulances and hospitals; viz., 50,000 for wounds, and 150,000 for diseases. The medical officers of the French army arranged their plans for taking care of their sick and wounded on the basis of the calculation that 10 per cent. would be under treatment at one time. So, at the period when the number of their troops was limited to 40,000, they made provision for 4,000 to 5,000 patients. In the attacks of cholera during the Dobrudscha expedition the proportion of deaths to attacks was as 1 to $1\frac{3}{10}$. More than 8,000 French soldiers were placed *hors du combat* by the cholera in the epidemic of Varna and Dobrudscha. At the end of February of the first winter in the Crimea, there were 3,000 cases of scurvy in the French army, averaging 100 for each old regiment, and 25 for each new one. At the same period the wounds presented an unhealthy appearance, the granulations were flabby, traumatic gangrene was frequently observed. In the month of June, 1855, there were 4,000 cases of cholera, and more than six thousand wounds. The medical officers suffered greatly in health from their incessant and exhausting labors, about one-third of their number being sick. After the battle of Traktir Bridge, in August, 1855, the French surgeons performed 300 amputations and resections. A number of them were obliged to walk a great distance to the field of action; they were occupied with dressing wounds nearly the whole day, exposed to the heat of the sun, and then returned in the afternoon to the stationary ambulances, to perform urgent operations, which were not completed before midnight. The Malakoff was taken in September, 1855, after 316 days of hard work and fighting in the trenches. A million of sand-bags and 80,000 gabions had been employed. There had been 600,000 discharges of cannon and mortars. Twenty leagues of trenches had been opened. After the taking of the Malakoff, the French surgeons had the care of 5,000 wounded persons, including many of the Russians. The whole number of patients under treatment at that time in the French ambulances was 10,520. In one division, three surgeons and one apothecary had the entire care of 900 patients. The number of the wounded after the battle of the Tchernaia was 2,474; viz., 810 French and 1,664 Russians, coming under the care of the French surgeons. Typhus fever broke out in the French army in December, 1855; in that month there were 734 cases. In January there were 1,523 cases. During the two months, 787 cases terminated fatally. In February there were 3,402 cases, of which 1,435 were fatal. The disease attacked large numbers of persons who had been previously sick with other diseases. Every other disease seemed to be transformed into this terrible scourge. Seventy-five French surgeons in the Crimea were sick with typhus, and thirty-one died of it. Scrive says that "the losses occasioned by the most murderous battles do not equal one-fourth of the total losses to which an army is ordinarily subjected." Scrive, in reporting the sanitary condition of the army in February, 1856, makes the following remarks: "The regiments were not all attacked in the same degree. The proportion of the sick bears a close relation to the energy of the exciting causes. Thus, but few patients were found in the 17th battalion of chasseurs—10 out of 450 men. This battalion is comfortably quartered in barracks of good elevation; the ground is carefully paved; each soldier has a bed raised thirty centimetres, or about twelve inches, from the ground. Perfect cleanliness is observed throughout. The sea of mud of the adjoining streets is replaced by a stone pavement. Great care is taken as to diet, and vegetables are never wanting. The chasseurs are a chosen body of robust and intelligent men, and the site of their encampment is a very healthy one. The 85th regiment is the worst treated of all; it counts about 200 patients, waiting until places can be found for them in the hospitals. This regiment is badly sheltered, and presents all the causes of disease in an exaggerated state. Among the other regiments, the 57th has nearly 200 sick, the 10th has 150, the 61st 200, the 6th dragoons 40, 7th dragoons 30, 4th hussars 50, infantry of marine 20, engineers 13, artillery 100. In all these regiments there is not a single case of sickness among the officers, who are better lodged and fed." The whole number of French troops sent to the army of the East, as already mentioned, was 309,268: the whole number of deaths was 69,229; of this number there were 7,500 who were killed on the battle-field, or not afterwards heard from. The total attacks of cholera in the French army of the East amounted to 18,400. Of this number 11,000 were fatal. Attacks 1 to 15 of the army; deaths 1 to $1\frac{6}{10}$ of the cases. The total attacks of typhus were about 35,000; total deaths from the same disease 17,515. The whole number of cases of diarrhœa was 19,339, of dysentery 6,105. Scurvy prevailed to a great extent during the severe cold of winter, and during the sultry heat of summer, but almost disappeared during the spring and autumn. Scrive says that "the single efficient cause of scurvy was the absence of fresh vegetables." He adds, "Scurvy, like typhus, can be created at will." A considerable number of French soldiers died from exposure to cold, frosted limbs, etc. Most of these were intemperate persons. Among the wounded in battle, 1 in 5 died on the field, the proportion being the same in the three battles of Alma, Inkerman, and Traktir Bridge. The proportion of amputations was about 1 out of 6 wounded. During the first five or six weeks of the siege the health of the troops was good, and the wounds pursued a favorable course; at a later period the wounds did not do so well.

From the facts which have been presented, it is very evident that the lives of military men are much more endangered by disease than by wounds received in battle. It is, then, one of the highest duties of an army surgeon to make himself well acquainted with the correct principles of military hygiene, and to exert his influence to the greatest possible extent in promoing the health and physical energy of the soldiers who are intrusted to his care. Your committee proposes to consider the subject of military hygiene in some of its most important details.

I. *The Selection of a Ground for an Encampment.*

It is a matter of the utmost importance, whenever it is practicable, to avoid encamping in a malarious district. The encamping ground should be dry, moderately elevated, and with a sufficient slope to prevent water from stagnating when it rains. It should be in the vicinity of pure water drinking and washing, and there should be an abundant supply of fuel for cooking. The want of water in the vicinity of an encampment is a very formidable evil. When the French army, after the battle of Alma, encamped near the village of Mackenzie, they found but two or three wells, which were soon exhausted. The soldiers called the camp "the camp of thirst." They endured great suffering in consequence of the want of water. In selecting a site for encampment on the banks of a river, care should be taken to guard against the danger of inundation by a rapid rise of the water, from melting of snow, or from a sudden fall of rain. If military necessity should require an encampment in the neighborhood of an extensive marsh, the ground should always, if possible, be selected on the windward side, so that the prevailing winds should carry away the noxious emanations from the soil. When soldiers are exposed to cold and damp air without suitable protection, the injurious effects of such exposure will be diminished by the judicious use of camp-fires. In malarious districts, the protective use of the sulphate of quinine is to be highly commended. Each man may take three to ten grains daily, according to the intensity of the malarious influence. It may be taken in one dose at bedtime.

II. *The Construction and Arrangement of Tents, and other means which are employed to protect the Soldiers from the Weather.*

Tents should be made of a strong material and of close texture, so as to perfectly exclude the rain. The ground on which the soldier lies should be covered with boards, with straw, with twigs of pine, hemlock, or cedar, or with india-rubber cloth, to exclude the moisture from beneath. In hot weather, where there are no shade-trees, the tents should be double, to exclude the solar heat, and ventilation should be afforded on the shady side. There should also be openings for ventilation at the upper part of the tents, to carry off the heated gases which accumulate in those regions. A sufficient number of tents should be provided to prevent over-crowding; and if, in any emergency, it should be necessary to crowd an unusual number of persons in a tent, the evil should be counterbalanced, as far as circumstances will permit, by increased ventilation. The tents should not be allowed to remain many days in the same position, as the ground which they cover absorbs the emanations from the body, and thus vitiates the air. In fine weather the tents should frequently be taken down in the morning and put up again in the afternoon or evening. Every fine day the clothing and bedding should be freely exposed to the outer air. A sufficient space should be allowed between the tents to admit free ventilation. When the tents have been removed to a new ground, unless it be to a great distance from their former site, the ground from which they have been removed should be purified by sprinkling it freely with charcoal, lime, or other disinfecting agents. When circumstances forbid the removal of the tents, the ground may be purified by a similar use of antiseptic agents. The French army surgeons in the Crimea used sulphate of iron as a disinfecting agent. It was dissolved in fifteen times its weight of water. Three litres were used to disinfect a square metre of ground. It was also poured on collections of filth. fæces, &c. A litre is a little more than a quart; a metre is about thirty-nine inches.

When soldiers are making forced marches, and means of rapid transportation are insufficient, as they usually are on such occasions, it is better to dispense with the use of tents, and to sleep in the open air, as a more abundant supply of food, clothing, blankets, and other articles which are more indispensable to the health and comfort of the troops, may thus be transported. When an army is to be encamped during the winter, wooden huts are to be preferred to tents, as affording better protection to their inmates. In the construction of these huts, it is very important to make ample provision for efficient ventilation, and to avoid over-crowding. There should be openings for ventilation at the ends, sides, and ridge of each hut They should also have projecting eaves—boards to protect the sides from the heat of the sun, and to prevent the entrance of rain or snow through the openings which are left for ventilation. They should be whitewashed with lime within and without. Care should be taken to prevent accumulations of water about tents or huts. The ground should be sloping, and, whenever it is necessary, trenches should be dug to carry off the water. When an encampment is to remain long in one place, and the ground is tenacious of moisture, the streets between the tents or huts should be paved.

III. *The Disposition of Excrements and Offal.*

Pits should be dug on the leeward side of the camp, and ordinarily at a distance of not less than two hundred yards. They should be at least four feet in depth, and the bottom should be covered with charcoal. Such offal as cannot be consumed by fire should be thrown into the pits each day, and then covered with charcoal and a few inches of earth. When the matter reaches within two feet of the surface, cover with charcoal, and fill up with earth a little above the level of the adjacent surface. No pit should be dug for such purposes near any source from which water is supplied to the camp. Dead animals and offensive offal should be buried immediately, at such a depth that at least three feet should intervene between their upper surface and the level of the ground. Before the pit is filled in, the carcass or offal should be covered with charcoal. Similar precautions should be observed in the interment of human bodies. After a severe engagement, attended with great loss of life, the bodies should be interred in trenches eight or ten feet in depth. When offensive emanations arise from the ground, in consequence of the decomposition of organized substances, the surface should be covered with deodorizing materials. The British sanitary inspectors in the Crimea recommended for this purpose a compound consisting of one part of peat charcoal, one part of quicklime, and four parts of sand or gravel. Mr. Scrive, medical inspector of the French army in the Crimea, recommended a solution of chloride of lime for the same purpose. He sometimes directed the solution of sulphate of iron to accomplish this object. He also directed the bodies of men and animals to be covered with a thick stratum of lime, after being buried at a proper depth.

IV. *Clothing.*

Flannel should be worn next to the skin. The clothing should be light, and should be so adjusted as not to interfere with the most perfect freedom of muscular action. Each soldier should be provided with one or more blankets, for protection during the night. The clothing should be washed and thoroughly dried as often as circumstances will permit. From the first of October to the end of May, each soldier should be provided with a thick overcoat to protect him from cold and stormy weather. The feet should be covered with stockings, and stout shoes with broad soles and low heels. The shoes should not be tight so as to pinch the feet, but they should not be excessively loose. Great care is required with fresh recruits, to prevent the feet from becoming sore. If the heel becomes slightly chafed, the part should be at once covered with adhesive plaster. For want of this simple precaution many soldiers have become disabled, and have thus fallen into the hands of the enemy, and in contests with savages, have lost their lives.

In hot weather, the heads of the soldiers should be protected by means of straw hats or of havelocks.

V. *Supply and Preparation of Food and Drinks.*

This is a subject of great importance to the health and efficiency of armies, and the neglect of which is apt to be followed by the most disastrous consequences. It is highly important not only that the supply of food should be ample, but that its quality should be good, and that it should be in such a form that it can be prepared for use as speedily and with as little labor as possible. Hard biscuit or pilot-bread may be furnished alternately with soft bread; and care should be taken to prevent the use of any bread of inferior quality. Butter and cheese may be added with the morning and evening meal, on which occasion coffee or tea should also be provided. The coffee which is furnished to the men should be already roasted and ground, so that it can be prepared with little labor. There should always be a sufficient allowance of sugar and milk. Where fresh milk cannot be obtained in sufficient quantities, solidified milk may be used as a substitute. There should be a regular allowance of meat and vegetables at dinner, whenever it is practicable to furnish them. Soldiers should not be confined for a long time to salted meat; but fresh meat should always be allowed whenever it can be obtained. The use of fresh vegetables is of very great importance as a means of guarding against scurvy. There are many herbs or weeds growing in the fields or by the roadsides, which can be employed for this purpose when better vegetables cannot be obtained. Thus, the French soldiers in the Crimea derived the greatest advantages from the use of dandelion (Leontodon Taraxacum), dressed with oil and vinegar, and eaten as a salad. Fruits should also be provided in their season, either in a fresh or dried state. When fresh vegetables cannot be obtained, their place may be in part supplied by the use of vegetables desiccated in a rarified atmosphere. There seems to be no good reason why soldiers should not be fed as well, under ordinary circumstances as the better class of laboring men at home. It would be very desirable that there should be at least one good cook for every company of soldiers, as the wholesomeness of their food depends very much on the manner in which it is prepared. General Scott is reported to have said, that a man who cannot make good bread is not fit to be captain of a company. An ample supply of good water, for drinking and cooking, is a matter of great importance to the health and comfort of soldiers. It would be well if every regiment were supplied with a distilling apparatus, by means of which the water of marshes or even of the ocean could be purified. Distilled water, agitated so as to mix with it a sufficient quantity of air, might often be substituted with great advantage for the impure and unwholesome water which soldiers are compelled to drink. Great care should be taken to guard against the excessive use of alcoholic drinks. It would be well for the young men in our armies to make no use of these beverages, except when they are prescribed for medicinal purposes.

There can be no reasonable doubt that the health of armies has been in many instances greatly impaired, and that multitudes of valuable lives have been lost, in consequence of the insufficient quantity or the bad quality of the food which has been furnished. The errors which have been committed in this respect have sometimes been due to mistakes at head-quarters, sometimes to a want of knowledge or of attention on the part of the commissaries of regiments, and sometimes to the knavery of contractors, who have committed wholesale murder by depriving the soldiers of the full supply of good food which they have engaged to furnish, and for which they have received ample compensation. It is not improbable that the Austrian army was defeated at Solferino in consequence of the soldiers being exhausted by long fasting, the Commissary General having appropriated to his own use the funds which were furnished him for the purpose of providing rations for the army. It is important that the rations of the soldiers should, under ordinary circumstances, be issued daily. When rations are distributed at one time for several days, there is often at first an unnecessary waste, in consequence of which the soldiers afterwards suffer from want, or supply themselves by plunder. With regard to the hard biscuit usually furnished to the soldiers as a part of their diet, M. Scrive says, that it should be made thinner and more friable, as by its thickness and hardness it irritates and inflames the gums. M. Scrive also says, that when fresh meat cannot be supplied to the army, it should be replaced by preserved meats and soups; and that salt beef should, as far as possible, be abandoned as an article of food for soldiers, especially in long campaigns and in distant regions, as it is very apt to become spoiled. Borden's meat-biscuit may be a valuable article of diet, when fresh meat cannot be obtained. When soldiers have long been confined to the use of salted and smoked provisions, and fresh meat is afterwards liberally supplied to them, they are very apt to be attacked with severe and often fatal dysentery. The precaution should therefore be adopted to furnish to the men at first a very limited supply of fresh meat; the quantity may be gradually increased, as they become accustomed to its use. The dysentery, occurring under these circumstances, is stated by Dr. Hewitt, formerly surgeon in the U. S. army, to be most readily cured by purging with sulphate of magnesia.

VI. As a means of preserving the health of soldiers, great care should be taken, as far as military necessities will allow, to avoid excessive and exhausting labor, and to allow ample time for sleep. There is no doubt that a large part of the mortality among the troops who were engaged in the Crimean war was owing to the perhaps unavoidable violation of these rules. The men were engaged in almost incessant labor, and their sleep was often disturbed, while, at the same time, they were exposed to the heat and cold, rain and snow, with very insufficient protection. Whenever it is necessary to have a large amount of labor performed, it is better, if practicable, to hire laborers, than to require an excessive amount of work from the soldiers.

Under the head of military therapeutics, are to be considered the preparations which are required for the practice of medicine and surgery under the peculiar circumstances attending the movements of armies, and the actual treatment of diseases and injuries occurring under those circumstances. In laborious marches, in obstinate and protracted sieges, in sudden and unexpected assaults, in severe and bloody engagements, the military surgeon is called in rapid succession to the treatment of large numbers of sick and wounded soldiers. There is no time for calm deliberation and careful preparation; he cannot send his prescriptions to an apothecary, nor can he send to a manufacturer for new instruments or apparatus. The few medicines, instruments, and dressings which he requires, must be at hand, or his patients must be deprived of the benefits which they would have derived from them. A wise foresight must therefore be exercised in providing such materials as are indispensable to the care of the sick and wounded, and in conveying them to every place where they may be needed. All bulky and heavy articles which are not absolutely essential should be dispensed with, on account of the difficulty and delay in conveying them from place to place. The best way of conveying the apparatus of an army surgeon is a box-cart, similar to those which are often used by peddlers. In going over a country too rough for wheel-carriages, a pair of panniers slung over the back of a horse or mule is the best substitute for a cart. The weight of the panniers with their contents should not exceed 200 lbs.

Each surgeon should be provided with a case of amputating and trephining instruments, with scalpels, bistouries, lancets, and other instruments for minor operations. He should always have about his person a good case of pocket instruments, and a canteen containing wine or brandy and water, ready to be used as a cordial in any case of emergency. He should also carry in his pocket a phial containing pills of opium. In the cart or panniers containing his apparatus there should be a supply of sponges, bandages, lint, tow, cotton batting, old linen or muslin for compresses, ligatures, tin basins, splints, adhesive plaster, pins, needles, matches, candles, catheters and bougies, a stomach pump, an enema pump, and a suppository syringe. There should be a dozen tourniquets, and the orderly men, who act as assistants to the surgeon, should be instructed in their application. There should also be a supply of anæsthetics and of medicines suitable to the emergencies of military life. On the field of battle, each surgeon should be immediately followed by an orderly man, bearing a knapsack containing a few of the most indispensable instruments and dressings for immediate use. Previously to an engagement, a certain number of men from each company should be deputed to take charge of such soldiers as may be wounded, and to remove them at once to a place of safety in the rear of the army. For this purpose, litters should be at hand, made of stout canvas, with stretchers, and provided with rings, into which bayonets or poles may be inserted. Ambulance carts should also be brought as near as possible to the scene of the engagement, and the wounded soldiers should be speedily deposited in them, and driven off to the place selected, where they may receive proper surgical attention.

The U. S. Army medical board recommend that the following schedule of transports for the sick and wounded, and for hospital supplies, be adopted for a state of war with a civilized enemy:

"For commands of less than three companies, one two-wheeled transport cart for hospital supplies; and to each company, one two-wheeled ambulance.

"For commands of more than three and less than five companics, two two-wheeled transport carts; and to each company, one two-wheeled ambulance.

"For a battalion of five companies, one four-wheeled ambulance, five two-wheeled ambulances, and two two-wheeled transport carts. For each additional company, less than ten, one two-wheeled transport cart.

"For a regiment of ten companies, two four-wheeled ambulances, ten two-wheeled ambulances, and four two-wheeled transport carts; and for greater commands in proportion."

Also that "horse-litters may be prepared and furnished to posts, whence they may be required for service on ground not admitting the employment of two-wheeled carriages; said litters to be composed of a canvas bed similar to the presents tretcher, and of two poles, each sixteen feet long, to be made in sections with head and foot pieces, constructed to act as stretchers to keep the poles apart."

Also, that "the allowance of hospital attendants in the field will be, for one company, one steward, one nurse, and one cook; for each additional company, one nurse; and for commands of over five companies, one additional cook."

The army Board also recommend hospital tents of the following dimensions: "In length, 14 feet; in width, 15 feet; in height (centre) 11 feet, with a wall 4½ feet, and a fly of appropriate size. The ridge pole to be made in two sections, and to measure 14 feet when joined." The Board contemplate that such a tent will accommodate 8 to 10 patients comfortably. It is evident, however, that the space allowed for each patient is altogether too small, amounting to only a little more than 160 cubic feet for each patient.

In making arrangements for the care of sick and wounded soldiers, there should be hospital tents erected as near as possible to the field of battle, so that dressings and operations which are urgently required, may be performed without any unnecessary delay. There should also be regimental hospitals, which may be constructed as tents, huts, or more permanent buildings, according to the season of the year and the character of the military operations. Each regimental hospital should have accommodations for fifty to one hundred patients. There should also be general hospitals at the base of operations, and in these there should be ample accommodations for all the patients which may be sent to them from the regimental hospitals, or directly from the camps or the battle-field. The regimental and general hospitals should contain sufficient space to allow not less than eight hundred cubic feet of air for each patient. The horizontal space should not be less than 6 by 6 feet for each patient. Large public buildings, such as churches, concert-rooms, and public halls, are commonly employed as general military hospitals. It is often necessary to make extensive alterations to adapt them to their new use. Special regard should be paid to ventilation. The doors and windows usually require to be enlarged, especially in an upward and downward direction; or numerous holes, six inches square, may be made through the walls near the floors and ceilings. There should be doors and windows opposite to each other, so as to allow the air to pass freely through in all directions. The patients should not be placed in stories below the level of the ground or but slightly raised above it, as experience has shown that the upper stories are much more salubrious. The beds should be raised from the floor, being placed on iron bedsteads whenever they can be obtained. No two bedsteads should be in contact, and none should touch the walls of the room. No unnecessary articles should be in the wards, as they occupy valuable space, and absorb noxious vapors. Care should be taken that the windows do not open upon any receptacles of foul air. Besides the principal hospital buildings, there should be small detached houses reserved for special cases. Near the entrance of the town some building or tents should be selected as receiving hospital, where the wounded should be brought and properly cleansed, wounds dressed, and suitable hospital clothes provided; and then they should be forwarded to the permanent hospital. Great attention should be paid to privies and drains connected with the hospital, to prevent them from contaminating the atmosphere. Patients who are able to rise from their beds should eat in adjoining rooms or tents. The wards of the hospitals should be divided into three classes, viz., surgical, medical, and convalescent. To every division of one hundred beds, there should be at least one ward superintendent and six orderly-men. When the hospital is prepared, the compound fractures should be placed in the most accessible wards, and injuries of the same character should be placed in the same wards. When wine or spirits are directed, the surgeon should see them administered. To preserve the purity of the air, the wards should be frequently whitewashed with lime. The adjacent grounds should be well drained, and the sewers should be frequently flushed. Excretions should be as soon as possible removed from the wards. The temporary hospitals attached to camps are subject to terrible mishaps. Bazancourt speaks in the following terms of the effects of a hurricane upon the frail structure used as a military hospital by the French army in the Crimea: "The ambulance barracks are shattered by the fury of the wind; and whilst their roofs, carried up in the air, whirl around and disappear, the broken timbers fall upon the wounded and the sick, whose beds are overturned into the pools of rain which inundate them. Most of the patients are unable to move, being quite prostrated by illness, or by severe wounds, and lie waiting with resignation that which the will of God may determine respecting them."

In the French army in the Crimea each ambulance for ten thousand men had three caissons, containing materials for six thousand dressings, and eighteen complete tents. Flying ambulances on mules' backs were provided for regions where carriages could not go. As an example of the manner of taking care of the wounded during and after an engagement, your Committee presents the following directions given by M. Scrive to the medical officers of the French army in June, 1855: "At the ambulance of the trenches shall be assembled before the battle the non-combatant soldiers—the musicians of the regiment, for example, with the infirmary men disposable in the different services. One or several officers of administration will direct them in the trenches to take up the wounded, and transport them to the ambulance. An officer of administration, having a fixed position at the ambulance, will attend to placing the wounded, on their arrival, in an order always the same, and determined beforehand to avoid confusion. The visits to the wounded shall be made by one or more surgeons, assisted by two or more infirmary men carrying dressings, &c.; one of these last will inscribe the name of the patient, his regiment, and his matriculated number. The surgeon will determine whether the wound requires to be dressed immediately, or if the patient can be at once transported to the ambulance of the division. In the first place, the wound may be dressed on the spot, or, if an immediate operation is required, the patient may be conveyed into the operating room. After the dressing or operation, the patient may be placed upon the litter or ambulance cart. Where four to six wounded persons are ready, they shall be conveyed together to the ambulance of the division; and in these little successive journeys, the muleteers, under the direction of an officer commanding the train, shall betake themselves to the ambulance, whose number shall have been designated by the military sub-intendant or his aid, who shall mark upon the list of vacant places, at the different stationary ambulances, the names of the wounded whom he will send there successively. In this manner the exact situation of the ambulances will be precisely known. When the wounded are very numerous, no operations shall be performed excepting those which are absolutely necessary. One-third of the surgeons shall be constantly occupied in visiting the wounded, and judging as to the necessity of immediate operation or dressing, especially when the number of the wounded is large; the remaining two-thirds shall attend to the necessary operations and dressings, following, except in cases of great urgency, the order of arrival and the rank of the patient. In the ambulance of the trenches, the services of the infirmary men may be conveniently divided in the following manner: two infirmary men for each surgeon engaged in dressing; two infirmary men for each surgeon on his visits—one to write, and the other to assist the patient to get on the litter; four infirmary men for an operating table; and finally, eight to twelve infirmary men engaged as porters, to attend to the transportation of the wounded. It is very important to prevent the crowding of the ambulance of the trenches by soldiers whose aid is not required. A guard should therefore be placed at the door to prevent such persons from entering. In the ambulance of the division, on the day of battle, two surgeons should be on duty to receive the wounded coming from the trenches, and to examine minutely each wound. They shall make a definitive dressing in cases where an immediate operation is not indicated."

The general practice of the French surgeons in the Crimea was to extract foreign bodies from wounds at an early period, whenever they were easily accessible. The most efficient styptics in arresting hemorrhage, where the blood-vessels could not be conveniently tied, were the perchloride and the persulphate of iron. Amputations were generally resorted to in severe injuries of the limbs, and the results were more favorable than when conservative surgery was attempted. Primary amputations were much more successful than secondary. Scrive makes an exception to this rule, in the case of amputation of the hip-joint. Nine primary amputations at this joint were performed by the French surgeons in the Crimea, and in all death took place within a few hours after the operation. There were three consecutive amputations at the hip: the patients severally lived five, twelve, and twenty days. Resections were generally fatal, except in the upper extremity. Scrive remarks, that when amputation was performed a day or two after an injury, it was much more difficult to induce anæsthesia than when the amputation was performed on the same day. The amputations were as follows: hip, 12; thigh, 1,512; knee, 58; leg, 915; foot, 241; toes, 220; shoulder, 168; arm, 912; elbow, forearm, and wrist, 278; hand and fingers, 282. The average dressings for each patient were: of linen, 2,482 grammes; roller bandages, 891 grammes; charpie, 1,181 grammes. The weight of dressings during the campaign amounted to 196,000 kilogrammes. (A gramme is about 15 grains; a kilogramme 2 lbs. 8 oz. troy weight). Average number of dressings for each wounded person, 35; total number of dressings, 1,400,000. Number of surgeons wounded by the fire of the enemy and by the explosion of magazine, 19. One died in consequence of his wounds. The labors of the surgeons were excessively severe. Each surgeon, on an average, was obliged to visit daily more than 100 patients. Eighty-three French army surgeons died during the war. It is very evident that the amount of labor thrown upon the medical officers of the French army was unreasonably great, and that the number of these officers should have been largely increased. When an army is called into active service, and is exposed to pestilential diseases and to bloody engagements, a much larger amount of medical service is required than can be reasonably expected of a surgeon and an assistant surgeon to each regiment.

Your Committee does not consider it necessary to enter into the details of the treatment which is required in gunshot wounds, and in other injuries to which soldiers are exposed, as these subjects are treated at considerable length in the textbooks of surgery, which are in the hands of most of our practitioners. There are, however, some practical lessons to which a passing allusion may be made with advantage. When the attention of an army surgeon is first directed to a number of wounded persons, who have been brought from the field of battle, it is important to determine the order in which his services should be rendered to them. In order that the greatest amount of effectual relief may be afforded, certain rules may be laid down for the guidance of the surgeon under these trying circumstances. The cases to which the first attention of the surgeon should be given are not those of so severe a character as to be almost necessarily fatal; nor, on the other hand, those which are comparatively slight and unattended with danger. But his first attention should be directed to injuries which are severe and dangerous, but which at the same time afford a good prospect of recovery. The cases most urgently requiring immediate treatment are those in which there is alarming hemorrhage, the source of which is not beyond the reach of surgical skill. The cases next in order of urgency, are those in which, from the shock of the injury, there is more or less prostration, requiring the use of cordials and stimulants. Then come the cases of compound fracture, some of these requiring amputation or resection, and others mechanical support to prevent distortion and the irritation arising from muscular spasm, causing spiculæ of bone to penetrate the soft parts. Next in order come the slighter cases of injury of the viscera, always attended with danger, but not necessarily fatal. After disposing of those cases which are more or less hopeful, the surgeon may direct his attention to the comfort and relief of the more severe injuries, in which a fatal result is almost certain to ensue. And lastly, he may attend to the minor operations and dressings in cases of injury which are not regarded as dangerous to life.

The result of primary amputations at the hip-joint is so uniformly disastrous, that, in the opinion of your Committee, these operations should be discarded from military surgery. If the patient should in any case recover from the shock of the terrible injury which seems to require so formidable an operation as amputation at the hip-joint, the operation may be performed consecutively with better prospect of success, without diverting the attention of the surgeon, at this period, from a more hopeful class of cases.

There is another subject which your Committee would bring to the notice of the surgical section of the Academy, viz., the injurious consequences resulting from the hasty removal of the sick and wounded by a discomfited and retreating army. Under these circumstances, your Committee would suggest the expediency of leaving the sick and wounded, with a sufficient number of medical attendants, to fall into the hands of the enemy as prisoners of war, in all cases in which there is a large number of patients whose lives would be greatly endangered by the removal, and in which reliance could be placed on the magnanimity of the victorious party. There might be a previous understanding between the belligerent parties, that hospital buildings, or tents, so abandoned, and surmounted by a flag of truce, or some other preconcerted signal, should be safe from attack.

There is another subject to which the attention of the section might have been directed at an earlier part of the report, viz., the importance of a thorough inspection of recruits who present themselves for admission into the army. The admission of sickly and feeble men into an army is an evil of the greatest magnitude, not merely depriving the government of the services of such individuals, but exerting an injurious influence upon the health, spirit, and efficiency of their comrades. Every recruit should therefore undergo a most thorough inspection, and if deficient in the physical qualities which are necessary for a soldier, he should without hesitation be rejected. A soldier should be a full grown man, and not a boy. The most eligible age for a recruit is twenty to twenty-five years. A soldier should be strictly temperate in his habits, as intemperance is one of the most fruitful sources of disease as well as of insubordination and of crime. He should have perfect sight and perfect hearing, as a failure in either of these senses would render him incompetent to perform the duties which are expected of a soldier. He should be sound in all his vital organs, and should have a good degree of muscular development. The medical inspector should examine the recruit, divested of his clothing, investigating the condition of every vital organ, testing the sight and hearing, and subjecting the head, trunk, and limbs to ocular inspection, and to manual palpation. The condition of the urinary organs should not be overlooked, and the candidate should be required to pass his urine in the presence of the inspector. A careful investigation should be instituted with reference to the existence of hernia or aneurism. Ulcers or cicatrices on the legs, varicose veins, corns, bunions, and inverted toe-nails, should lead to the rejection of the candidate. If the inspection of recruits were more thoroughly conducted than it usually is, it would greatly add to the vigor and efficiency of our armies.

All which is respectfully submitted.

Alfred C. Post, M. D.,
Wm. H. Van Buren, M. D.,
Committee.

New York, *June* 21, 1861.

CPSIA information can be obtained
at www.ICGtesting.com
Printed in the USA
BVHW041534011218
534322BV00039B/256/P

9 780331 069556